BEST SALAD RECIPES 2022

EASY RECIPES FOR BEGINNERS

PETE COURIER

Table of Contents

Fatoosh 9

Tangy Pear and Blue Cheese Salad 11

Spicy Italian Salad 13

Caesar Salad II 15

Salad with Prosciutto and Caramelized Pears and Walnuts 17

Romaine and Mandarin Orange Salad with Poppy Seed Dressing 19

House Salad Restaurant-Style 21

Spinach Salad 23

Super Seven Spinach Salad 25

Beautiful Salad 26

Spinach and Orzo Salad 27

Strawberry, Kiwi, and Spinach Salad 29

Spinach Pomegranate Salad 30

Spinach Salad with Pepper Jelly Dressing 31

Super Easy Spinach and Red Pepper Salad 32

Spinach Watermelon-Mint Salad 33

Pretty Pomegranate Salad 35

Apple Almond Crunch Salad 36

Mandarin Orange, Gorgonzola and Almond Delight 37

Tossed Romaine and Orange Salad 38

Addicting Salad 39

Kale Salad with Pomegranate, Sunflower Seeds and Sliced Almonds .. 41

Pomegranate Feta Salad with Lemon Dijon Vinaigrette 43

Arugula, Fennel, and Orange Salad 45

Avocado Watermelon Spinach Salad 46

Avocado, Kale and Quinoa Salad.. 47

Zucchini Salad with Special Dressing 49

Vegetable and Bacon Salad 51

Crunchy Cucumber Salad 53

Colorful Veggie and Cheese Salad 54

Creamy Cucumber Salad... 56

Bacon and Broccoli Salad 58

Vegetables and Corn Bread Salad 60

Bean and Vegetable Salad 62

Corn and Olive Salad 64

Corn Salad 66

Fresh Hungarian Salad 68

A perfect mixture of tomato, cucumber and onion 70

Classic Cucumber Salad 72

Tomato Salad with Cherry Splash 74

Asparagus Salad 76

Pasta and Black Eyed Peas in Salad 78

Spinach and Beetroot Salad 80

Potato Salad with Balsamic Vinegar... 82

Marinated Tomato Salad 84

Tasty Broccoli Salad 86

Corn Salad with Italian Dressing 88

Asparagus and Bell Pepper Salad 89

Tomato and Basil Salad 91

Colorful Garden Salad... 93

Mushrooms Salad... 95

Quinoa, Mint and Tomato Salad	97
Sauerkraut Salad Recipe	99
Quick Cucumber Salad	101
Tomato Slices with Creamy Dressing	103
Beet Salad Platter	104
Chicken and Spinach Salad	106
German Cucumber Salad	108
Colorful Citrus Salad with Unique Dressing	110
Potato, Carrot and Beet Salad	112
Chicken Satay Healthier Healthy Salad Sammies	113
Cleopatra's Chicken Salad	115
Thai-Vietnamese salad	117
Christmas Cobb Salad	119
Green Potato Salad	122
Burnt corn salad	125
Cabbage and grape salad	127
Citrus salad	129
Fruit and lettuce salad	131
Apple and lettuce salad	133
Bean and capsicum salad	135
Carrot and dates salad	137
Creamy pepper dressing for salad	138
Hawaiian Salad	140
Burnt corn salad	142
Cabbage and grape salad	144
Citrus salad	146
Fruit and lettuce salad	148

Curry chicken salad	150
Strawberry spinach salad	152
Sweet restaurant slaw	154
Classic macaroni salad	156
Roquefort pear salad	158
Barbie's tuna salad	160
Holiday chicken salad	162
Mexican bean salad	164
Bacon ranch pasta salad	166
Red skinned potato salad	168
Black bean and couscous salad	170
Greek chicken salad	172
Fancy chicken salad	174
Fruity curry chicken salad	176
Wonderful chicken curry salad	178
Spicy carrot salad	180
Asian apple slaw	182
Squash and orzo salad	184
Salad with Watercress-fruit	186
Caesar Salad	188
Chicken Mango Salad	190
Orange salad with mozzarella	192
Three-bean salad	194
Miso tofu salad	196
Japanese radish Salad	198
Southwestern Cobb	200
Pasta Caprese	202

Smoked-Trout Salad 204

Egg salad with Beans 206

Ambrosia Salad 207

Wedge salad 209

Spanish pimiento salad 211

Mimosa salad 213

Classic Waldorf 215

Black eyed pea salad 217

Fatoosh

Ingredients:

Change Servings

2 Pita breads

8 Leaves romaine lettuce, torn into bite-size pieces

2 Green onions, chopped

1 Cucumber, chopped

3 Tomatoes cut into wedges

1 clove Garlic, peeled and chopped

2 tbsp. Sumac powder

¼ cup Lemon juice

¼ cup Olive oil

1 tsp. Salt

¼ tsp. Ground black pepper

¼ cup Chopped mint leaves

Method

Preheat oven to 350 degrees F, 175 degrees C . Toast pitas for 5 to 10 minutes in the preheated oven, until crisp. Break into bite size pieces. In a large bowl, mix together pita toasted pieces, and green onions, romaine lettuce, cucumber, and tomatoes. Serve immediately.

Enjoy!

Tangy Pear and Blue Cheese Salad

Ingredients

1/3 cup ketchup

½ cup distilled white vinegar

¾ cup white sugar

2 tsp. Salt

1 cup canola oil

2 heads romaine lettuce, chopped

4 ounces Crumbled blue cheese

2 Pears, Peeled, cored and chopped

½ cup Toasted chopped walnuts

½ Red onion, chopped

Method

In a small bowl, ketchup, sugar, vinegar, and salt are well combined. Gradually pour in oil, stirring constantly, until well blended. In a large serving bowl, toss together the lettuce, blue cheese, pears, walnuts, and red onion. Pour dressing over salad and toss to coat.

Enjoy!

Spicy Italian Salad

Ingredients:

½ cup Canola oil

1/3 cup Tarragon vinegar

1 tbsp. White sugar

1 Red bell pepper, cut into strips

1 Grated carrot

1 Thinly sliced red onion

¼ cup Black olives

¼ cup Pitted green olives

½ cup Sliced cucumber

2 tbsp. Grated Romano cheese

Ground black pepper to taste

Method

In a medium container mix the canola oil, sugar, dry mustard, thyme and garlic in a bowl. In a large bowl, toss together lettuce, red bell pepper, carrot, red onion, artichoke hearts, black olives, green olives, cucumber, and Romano cheese. Place in the refrigerator for 4 hours, or overnight. Season with pepper and salt. Serve chilled.

Enjoy!

Caesar Salad II

Ingredients:

1 head romaine lettuce

2 cups Croutons

1 Juiced lemon

1 Dash Worcestershire sauce

6 cloves garlic, minced

1 tbsp. Dijon mustard

½ cup Olive oil

¼ cup Parmesan Grated cheese

Method

Crush the croutons in a deep mixing bowl .Set aside. Mix the mustard, lemon juice and Worcestershire sauce in a bowl. Blend thoroughly in a mixer and slowly add olive oil until creamy. Pour dressing over the lettuce. Add the croutons and cheese and toss well. Serve immediately.

Enjoy!

Salad with Prosciutto and Caramelized Pears and Walnuts

Ingredients:

2 cups orange juice

2 tbsp. Red wine vinegar

2 tbsp. finely chopped red onion

1 tbsp. White sugar

1 tbsp. White wine

1 cup Walnut halves

½ cup White sugar

¼ cup Water

¾ cup virgin Extra olive oil

1 tbsp. Butter

2 Pears - peeled, cored and cut into wedges

Prosciutto, cut into thin strips-1/4 pound

2 Romaine hearts, rinsed and torn

Method

In a medium saucepan, first heat orange juice over medium-high heat, whisking often, until it is reduced by 1/4. Add to a blender, along with the vinegar, onion, sugar, wine, salt and pepper. Melt butter in a non-stick skillet over medium heat while blending on a low speed, remove cap and slowly drizzle in the olive oil to emulsify the dressing. Add sugar and water and cook, stirring constantly. Sauté pears and nuts in butter for 3 minutes. Remove from heat and set aside to cool. Add vinaigrette. Now, serve on a large Italian platter.

Enjoy!

Romaine and Mandarin Orange Salad with Poppy Seed Dressing

Ingredients:

6 Slices bacon

1/3 cup Apple cider vinegar

¾ cup White sugar

½ cup Red coarsely chopped onion

½ tsp. Dry mustard powder

¼ tsp. Salt

½ cup Vegetable oil1 tsp. Poppy seeds

10 cups Torn romaine lettuce leaves

10 ounces Mandarin drained orange segments

¼ cup Toasted slivered almonds

Method

Brown the bacon in a skillet. Drain, crumble and set aside. Place vinegar, sugar, red onion, mustard powder, and salt into the bowl of a blender. Reduce blender speed to medium-low. Stir in the poppy seeds, now blend until incorporated and the dressing is creamy. Toss the romaine with the crumbled bacon and Mandarin oranges in a large bowl. Top with the dressing and serve immediately.

Enjoy!

House Salad Restaurant-Style

Ingredients:

Change Servings

1 Romaine Large head lettuce- rinsed, dried and torn into pieces

4 ounces Jar pimento diced peppers, drained

2/3 cup Extra virgin olive oil

1/3 cup Red wine vinegar

1 tsp. Salt

1 Large head iceberg - rinsed, dried and torn into pieces

14 ounces Artichoke hearts, drained and quartered

1 cup Sliced red onion

¼ tsp. Ground black pepper

2/3 cup cheese - grated Parmesan

Method

Combine all the ingredients in a bowl and toss well. Serve immediately.

Enjoy!

Spinach Salad

Ingredients:

Change Servings

½ cup White sugar

1 cup Vegetable oil

2 tbsp. Worcestershire sauce

1/3 cup Ketchup

½ cup White vinegar

1 Small chopped onion

1 pound spinach - rinsed, dried and torn into bite size pieces

4 ounces Sliced water drained chestnuts

5 Slices bacon

Method

Combine all the ingredients in a bowl and toss well. Serve immediately.

Enjoy!

Super Seven Spinach Salad

Ingredients:

6 ounces Package baby spinach leaves

1/3 cup Cubed Cheddar cheese

1 Peeled, cored and diced Fuji apple

1/3 cup Finely chopped red onion

¼ cup Sweetened dried cranberries

1/3 cup Blanched slivered almonds

3 tbsp. Poppy seed salad dressing

Method

Combine all the ingredients in a bowl and toss well. Serve immediately.

Enjoy!

Beautiful Salad

Ingredients:

8 cups Baby spinach leaves

11 ounces Can mandarin drained oranges

½ Medium red onion, separately sliced into rings

1 cup feta Crumbled cheese

1 cup vinaigrette Balsamic salad dressing

1 ½ cups Sweetened dried cranberries

1 cup Honey-roasted sliced almonds

Method

Combine all the ingredients in a bowl and toss well. Serve immediately.

Enjoy!

Spinach and Orzo Salad

Ingredients:

16 ounces Package uncooked orzo pasta

10 ounces Package finely chopped baby spinach leaves

½ pound Crumbled feta cheese

½ Red nicely chopped onion

¾ cup Pine nuts

½ tsp. Dried basil

¼ tsp. Ground white pepper

½ cup Olive oil

½ cup Balsamic vinegar

Method

Bring a large pot of lightly salted water to a boil. Transfer to a large bowl and stir in spinach, feta, onion, pine nuts, basil and white pepper. Add orzo and cook for 8 to 10 minutes, drain and rinse with cold water. Toss with olive oil and balsamic vinegar. Refrigerate and serve cold.

Enjoy!

Strawberry, Kiwi, and Spinach Salad

Ingredients:

2 tbsp. Raspberry vinegar

2 ½ tbsp. Raspberry jam

1/3 cup Vegetable oil

8 cups Spinach, rinsed and torn into bite-size pieces

½ cup Chopped walnuts

8 Quartered strawberries

2 Peeled and sliced kiwis

Method

Combine all the ingredients in a bowl and toss well. Serve immediately.

Enjoy!

Spinach Pomegranate Salad

Ingredients:

1, 10 ounce bag baby spinach leaves, rinsed and drained

1/4 red onion, sliced very thin

1/2 cup walnut pieces

1/2 cup crumbled feta

1/4 cup alfalfa sprouts, optional

1 pomegranate, peeled and seeds separated

4 tbsp. balsamic vinaigrette

Method

Place spinach in a salad bowl. Top with red onion, walnuts, feta, and sprouts. Sprinkle pomegranate seeds over the top, and drizzle with vinaigrette.

Enjoy!

Spinach Salad with Pepper Jelly Dressing

Ingredients:

3 tbsp. Mild pepper jelly

2 tbsp. Olive oil

1/8 tsp. Salt

2 cups Baby spinach leaves

2 ounces Sliced goat cheese

1/8 tsp. Dijon mustard

Method

Combine all the ingredients in a bowl and toss well. Serve immediately.

Enjoy!

Super Easy Spinach and Red Pepper Salad

Ingredients:

¼ cup Olive oil

6 ounces Package baby spinach

½ cup cheese - grated Parmesan

¼ cup Rice vinegar

1 Red bell chopped pepper

Method

Combine all the ingredients in a bowl and toss well. Serve immediately.

Enjoy!

Spinach Watermelon-Mint Salad

Ingredients:

1 tbsp. Poppy seeds

¼ cup White sugar10 ounces Bag baby spinach leaves

1 cup Apple cider vinegar

¼ cup Worcestershire sauce

½ cup Vegetable oil

1 tbsp. Sesame seeds

2 cups Cubed seeded watermelon

1 cup Finely chopped mint leaves

1 Small thinly sliced red onion

1 cup Chopped toasted pecans

Method

Combine all the ingredients in a bowl and toss well. Serve immediately.

Enjoy!

Pretty Pomegranate Salad

Ingredients:

10 ounces Can drained mandarin oranges

10 ounces baby spinach leaves

10 ounces Arugula leaves

1 Peeled pomegranate and seeds separated

½ Red thinly sliced onion

Method

Combine all the ingredients in a bowl and toss well. Serve immediately.

Enjoy!

Apple Almond Crunch Salad

Ingredients:

10 ounces Package mixed salad greens

½ cup Slivered almonds

½ cup Crumbled feta cheese

1 cup Tart chopped and cored apple

¼ cup Sliced red onion

¼ cup Golden raisins

1 cup Raspberry vinaigrette salad dressing

Method

Combine all the ingredients in a bowl and toss well. Serve immediately.

Enjoy!

Mandarin Orange, Gorgonzola and Almond Delight

Ingredients:

½ cup Blanched slivered almonds, dry roasted

1 cup Gorgonzola cheese

2 tbsp. Red wine vinegar

11 ounces Mandarin oranges, juice reserved

2 tbsp. Vegetable oil

12 ounces mixed salad greens

Method

Combine all the ingredients in a bowl and toss well. Serve immediately.

Enjoy!

Tossed Romaine and Orange Salad

Ingredients:

½ cup Orange juice

1 romaine large head lettuce - torn, washed and dried

3 cans Mandarin oranges

½ cup Slivered almonds

3 tbsp. Olive oil

2 tbsp. Red wine vinegar

½ tsp. Ground black pepper

¼ tsp. Salt

Method

Combine all the ingredients in a bowl and toss well. Serve immediately.

Enjoy!

Addicting Salad

Ingredients:

1 cup Mayonnaise

½ cup freshly grated cheese

½ cup Grated carrot

¼ cup freshly cheese - grated Parmesan

2 tbsp. White sugar

10 ounces Package spring lettuce mix

½ cup Small cauliflower florets

½ cup Bacon bits

Method

In a small bowl, 1/4 cup Parmesan cheese, and sugar, mayonnaise are combined together until they are properly blended. Cover, then keep it to refrigerate overnight. Combine the lettuce, bacon bits, 1/2 cup carrot, Parmesan cheese, cauliflower in a large serving bowl. Mix with chilled dressing just before serving.

Enjoy!

Kale Salad with Pomegranate, Sunflower Seeds and Sliced Almonds

Ingredients:

½ pound Kale

1 ½ cups Pomegranate seeds

5 tbsp. Balsamic vinegar

3 tbsp. extra virgin olive oil

2 tbsp. Sunflower seeds

1/3 cup Slivered almonds

5 tbsp. Red pepper seasoned rice vinegar

Salt to taste

Method

Wash and shake off extra water from the kale. Chop the leaves until fine but still a little leafy. The sliced almonds, chopped kale, pomegranate seeds, and sunflower seeds are mixed in a large bowl; toss to combine. Remove the center ribs and stems. The olive oil, rice vinegar, balsamic vinegar mixture is sprayed over the kale mixture and tossed. It is seasoned with salt to serve.

Enjoy!

Pomegranate Feta Salad with Lemon Dijon Vinaigrette

Ingredients:

10 ounces Package mixed baby greens

8 ounces Package crumbled feta cheese

1 Zested and juiced lemon

1 tsp. Dijon mustard

1 Peeled pomegranate and seeds separated

3 tbsp. Red wine vinegar

3 tbsp. Extra-virgin olive oil

Salt and pepper to taste

Method

The lettuce, feta cheese, and pomegranate seeds are placed into a large mixing bowl. Then, the lemon juice and zest, vinegar, mustard, salt, olive oil and pepper are whisked together in a large separate bowl. The mixture is poured over the salad and toss to coat. Now serve immediately to dig in.

Enjoy!

Arugula, Fennel, and Orange Salad

Ingredients:

½ tsp. Ground black pepper

¼ cup Olive oil

1 bunch Arugula

1 tbsp. Honey

1 tbsp. Lemon juice

½ tsp. Salt

2 Peeled and segmented orange

1 bulb thinly sliced fennel bulb

2 tbsp. Sliced black olives

Method

Combine all the ingredients in a large bowl and toss well. Serve immediately. Enjoy!

Avocado Watermelon Spinach Salad

Ingredients:

2 Large peeled, pitted and diced avocados

4 cups Cubed watermelon

4 cups spinach leaves

1 cup vinaigrette Balsamic salad dressing

Method

Combine all the ingredients in a large bowl and toss well. Serve chilled.

Enjoy!

Avocado, Kale and Quinoa Salad

Ingredients

2/3 cup Quinoa

1 bunch Kale cut bite-sized pieces

½ Avocado, peeled and diced

1/3 cup Red bell pepper, chopped

½ cup Cucumber, cut into small cubes

2 tbsp. Red onion, finely chopped

1 1/3 cups Water

1 tbsp. Crumbled feta cheese

For Dressing

¼ cup Olive oil2 tbsp. Lemon juice

1 ½ tbsp. Dijon mustard

¾ tsp. Sea salt

¼ tsp. Black pepper, freshly grounded

Method

Add quinoa and water in a saucepan. Bring it to boil. Reduce the flame and cook 15 to 20 minutes. Keep it aside. Steam the kale using a steamer for 45 second. Whisk all the ingredients for seasoning in a bowl. Mix kale, quinoa, avocado, and the rest items and top it with salad dressing.

Enjoy!

Zucchini Salad with Special Dressing

Ingredients

6 Small zucchini, sliced thinly

½ cup Green pepper, chopped

½ cup Onion, diced

½ cup Celery, diced

1 jar Pimientos, drained and diced

2/3 cup Vinegar

3 tbsp. White wine vinegar

1/3 cup Vegetable oil

½ cup Sugar

½ tsp. Pepper

½ tsp. Salt

Method

Mix all the vegetables in a medium sized bowl and keep aside. Mix all other ingredients in a jar with tight cover. Shake the mixture vigorously and pour it over the vegetables. Toss the veggies gently. Cover and keep it in the refrigerator overnight or minimum 8 hours. Served chilled.

Enjoy!

Vegetable and Bacon Salad

Ingredients

3 cups chopped broccoli

3 cups chopped cauliflower

3 cups chopped celery

6 slices bacon

1 ½ cups mayonnaise

¼ cup Parmesan cheese

1 package frozen green peas, defrosted

1 cup sweetened dried cranberries

1 cup Spanish peanuts

2 tbsp. grated onion

1 tbsp. white wine vinegar

1 tsp. salt

¼ cup white sugar

Method

Cook bacon in a large, deep skillet until they become nicely brown. Place it on the plate and crumble. In a large bowl, mix the broccoli, cauliflower, peas, cranberries and celery together. In another bowl, mix the cheese, mayonnaise, onion, sugar, vinegar and salt together. Pour the mixture over the vegetables. Throw nuts, bacon and toss it well. Serve immediately or chilled.

Enjoy!

Crunchy Cucumber Salad

Ingredients

2 quarts Small cucumbers, sliced with its peel

2 Onions, thinly sliced

1 cup Vinegar

1 ¼ cups Sugar

1 tbsp. Salt

Method

Mix onion, cucumber and salt in a bowl and allow it to soak for 3 hours. Take a saucepan and add vinegar and warm it. Add sugar to it and stir the mixture continuously till the sugar gets dissolved. Remove the cucumber from the soaked mixture and drain extra liquid. Add cucumber into the vinegar mixture and mix it. Put the mixture into plastic freezer bags or container. Freeze it. Defrost and serve it chilled.

Enjoy!

Colorful Veggie and Cheese Salad

Ingredients

1/3 cup Red or green bell pepper, diced

1 cup Celery, diced

1 packet Frozen green peas

3 Sweet pickles, finely chopped

6 Lettuce

2/3 cup Mayonnaise ¾ cup Cheddar cheese, cut into cubes

Pepper, freshly grounded

Salt to taste

Method

Take a large bowl. Mix mayonnaise, pepper, and salt together. Add red or green bell pepper, pickles, celery, and peas to the mixture. Combine all the ingredients well. Add cheese to the mixture. Chill it for 1 hour. Place the lettuce leaves on the salad dish and pile the mixture on the leaves.

Enjoy!

Creamy Cucumber Salad

Ingredients

9 cups Cucumbers, peeled and thinly sliced,

8 Green onions, finely chopped

¼ tsp. Onion salt

¼ tsp. Garlic salt

½ cup Yogurt

½ cup Low fat mayonnaise

¼ tsp. Pepper

2 drops Hot pepper sauce

¼ cup Evaporated milk

¼ cup Cider vinegar

¼ cup Sugar

Method

Take a large bowl. Place the cucumber, green onions, onion salt, garlic salt, and yogurt in a bowl and mix it well. Combine mayonnaise, pepper, pepper sauce, milk, vinegar, sugar and form a homogenous mixture. Spread the dressing over the cucumber mixture. Toss it well so that all the veggies get coated with the dressing. Refrigerate the salad for 4 hours. Serve it chilled.

Enjoy!

Bacon and Broccoli Salad

Ingredients

1 head broccoli, sliced into bite size pieces

10 slices Bacon

¼ cup Red onion, finely chopped

½ cup Raisins

3 tbsp. White wine vinegar

1 cup Mayonnaise

1 cup Sunflower seeds

2 tbsp. White sugar

Method

Take a large skillet. Cook the bacon till it gets evenly brown. Crumble and keep it aside. Place the broccoli, raisins and onion in a bowl and toss the mixture. Take a small bowl and whisk together the mayonnaise, vinegar, and sugar. Transfer it to the broccoli mixture and toss. Refrigerate for two hours. Before serving, add bacon and sunflower seed.

Enjoy!

Vegetables and Corn Bread Salad

Ingredients

1 cup Corn bread, coarsely crumbled

1 can Whole kernel corn, drained

½ cup Onion, chopped

½ cup Cucumber, chopped

½ cup Broccoli, chopped

½ cup Green pepper and sweet red pepper, chopped finely

½ cup Seeded tomato, chopped

½ cup Peppercorns

Ranch salad dressing

Salt & pepper to taste

Lettuce leaves

Method

Take a large bowl. Add the corn bread and veggies. Toss the mixture. Sprinkle salad dressing over the mixture. Add salt and pepper according to your taste. Toss it again. Cover the mixture and refrigerate it for a minimum of 4 hours. Put the salad on the lettuce leaves and serve.

Enjoy!

Bean and Vegetable Salad

Ingredients

2 cans whole kernel corn, drained

1 can black beans, rinsed and drained

8 green onions, finely chopped

2 jalapeno peppers, de-seeded and finely chopped

1 green bell pepper, thinly sliced

1 avocado, peeled and diced

1 jar pimentos

3 tomatoes, sliced

1/2 cup Italian salad dressing

1/2 tsp. garlic salt

1 cup chopped cilantro

1 lime, juiced

Method

Mix the black beans and corn in a large bowl. Add green onions, bell pepper, jalapeno peppers, pimentos, avocado, and tomatoes and toss the mixture. Add cilantro, lime juice and Italian dressing over the mixture. Add garlic salt for seasoning. Toss it well. Serve it chilled.

Enjoy!

Corn and Olive Salad

Ingredients

1 packet Frozen corn

3 Hard-cooked eggs

½ cup Mayonnaise

1/3 cup Pimiento-stuffed olives

2 tbsp. Chives, minced

½ tsp. Chili powder

¼ tsp. Ground cumin

1/8 tsp. Salt

Method

Combine the corn, sliced eggs and olives in a large bowl. Mix the mayonnaise and other ingredients for seasonings in a medium sized bowl. Add the mayonnaise to the corn mixture. Stir it well so that all the vegetables and corn get coated with the mayonnaise. Cover the bowl. Refrigerate it for 2 hours. Serve chilled.

Enjoy!

Corn Salad

Ingredients

6 Corns, husked, washed and drained

3 large Tomatoes

1 Onion, thinly sliced

¼ cup basil, minced

2 tbsp. White vinegar

¼ cup Olive oil

Salt & pepper to taste

Method

Cook the corns in a pan of boiling water and drain them and keep aside to cool. Cut the kernels off the cob. Take a large salad mixing bowl. Mix corn, basil, onion, tomatoes, vinegar, salt and pepper, and oil. Toss it well. Served chilled.

Enjoy!

Fresh Hungarian Salad

Ingredients

1 package frozen mixed vegetables, defrosted

1 cup cauliflowers

1/2 cup sliced green onions

1/2 cup sliced pimiento-stuffed olives

1/4 cup canola oil

3 tbsp. white vinegar

1/4 tsp. pepper

1 tsp. garlic salt

Method

Combine frozen vegetables, cauliflower, onion, and olives in a large bowl. Blend the oil, garlic salt, vinegar, and pepper in the blender. Pour the salad dressing over the vegetable mixture. Toss it well. Refrigerate for 2 hours before serve. Serve it in a nice bowl.

Enjoy!

A perfect mixture of tomato, cucumber and onion

Ingredients

2 large cucumber, halved and de-seeded

1/3 cup red wine vinegar

1 tbsp. white sugar

1 tsp. salt

3 large chopped tomatoes

2/3 cup coarsely chopped red onion

Method

Combine all the ingredients together and refrigerate overnight. Serve chilled.

Enjoy!

Classic Cucumber Salad

Ingredients

2 large cucumbers, peeled and sliced

1 large sweet onion, sliced

2 tsp. salt

¼ cup minced carrot

1/3 cup of vinegar

1 tsp. ground ginger

5 tsp. white sugar

¼ tsp. coarse black pepper

Method

Combine all the ingredients together and let the cucumber marinate in the fridge overnight. Serve chilled.

Enjoy!

Tomato Salad with Cherry Splash

Ingredients

4 cups halved cherry tomatoes

¼ cup vegetable oil

3 tbsp. cider vinegar

1 tsp. dried

1 tsp. dried basil

1 tsp. dried oregano

½ tsp. salt

1 tsp. white sugar

Method

Combine all the ingredients in a bowl and set aside so that the tomatoes soften a bit. Toss well and serve immediately.

Enjoy!

Asparagus Salad

Ingredients

1 ½ pounds asparagus, trimmed and sliced into 2-inch pieces

1 tbsp. Rice vinegar

1 tsp. Red wine vinegar

1 tsp. Soy sauce

1 tsp. White sugar

1 tsp. Dijon mustard

2 tbsp. Peanut oil

1 tbsp. Sesame oil

1 tbsp. Sesame seeds

Method

Put the rice vinegar, soy sauce, red wine vinegar, sugar, and mustard in a covered jar and mix well. Add the peanut oil as well as sesame oil slowly, continuously whisking it until smooth. Keep it aside. Cook the asparagus in boiling water and drain them. Place the asparagus in a large sized bowl. Sprinkle the salad dressing over them. Sprinkle sesame seeds and toss. Serve immediately.

Enjoy!

Pasta and Black Eyed Peas in Salad

Ingredients

6 ounces Cooked and drained small shell pasta

1 can Rinsed and drained black eyed peas

1 cup Sliced green onions

¾ cup Diced, peeled cucumber

¾ cup Diced tomato

¾ cup Diced green pepper

1 small jalapeno pepper, finely chopped

For Dressing:

3 tbsp. Canola oil

¼ cup Red wine vinegar

1 tsp. Dried basil

1 tsp. Hot pepper sauce

1 tsp. Chili powder

1 tsp. Sugar

½ tsp. Seasoned salt

Method

Combine pasta, peas, green onion, cucumber, tomato, green pepper and jalapeno pepper together in the bowl. Mix the dressing and season it with salt. Sprinkle the dressing over the vegetable mixture. Toss it well. Served it chilled.

Enjoy!

Spinach and Beetroot Salad

Ingredients

½ pound Baby spinach, washed and dried

1 cup Walnuts, chopped coarsely

2 ½ tbsp. White sugar

1/3 can pickled beets

¼ cup Cider vinegar

½ tsp. Garlic powder

1 tsp. Chicken bouillon granules

4 ounces Goat cheese, crushed

½ tsp. Black pepper

½ tsp. Salt

¼ cup Vegetable oil

Method

Caramelize the walnuts in a sauce pan, by heating them along with some sugar on high heat. Process the beets with cider vinegar, garlic powder, bouillon granules, salt, rest of the sugar, and pepper in a food processor. Pour oil and mix it again until smooth. Combine the sugar coated walnuts and spinach and sprinkle the dressing into it. Sprinkle cheese and serve immediately.

Enjoy!

Potato Salad with Balsamic Vinegar

Ingredients

10 Red potatoes, boiled and cubed

1 Onion, thinly sliced

1 can Quartered artichoke hearts

½ cup Red peppers, roasted then diced

1 can Black olives

½ cup Balsamic vinegar

1 tsp. Dried oregano

1 tsp. Dried basil

½ tsp. Mustard powder

3 tsp. Olive oil

2 tbsp. Fresh parsley

Method

Combine all the ingredients together in a bowl and toss well so that all the ingredients get coated with the vinegar. Refrigerate for 2-4 hours. Serve chilled.

Enjoy!

Marinated Tomato Salad

Ingredients

3 Tomatoes

2 tbsp. Chopped onion

1 tbsp. Fresh basil

1 tbsp. Fresh parsley

½ clove Garlic

1/3 cup olive oil

1/4 cup red wine vinegar

1/4 tsp. pepper

Salt to taste

Method

Take a nice large dish and place the tomatoes on it. Take a covered jar and put the vinegar, olive oil, basil, parsley, minced garlic and pepper in it and shake it vigorously, so that all the ingredients get combined well. Season the mixture with a pinch of salt or as per your taste. Pour the mixture over the tomatoes. Cover it properly and refrigerate overnight or for a minimum of 4 hours. Served chilled.

Enjoy!

Tasty Broccoli Salad

Ingredients

1 ½ pounds Fresh broccoli, cut into florets

3 cloves Garlic

2 tbsp. Lemon juice

2 tbsp. Rice vinegar

½ tsp. Dijon mustard

Red pepper flakes to taste

1/3 cup Olive oil

Salt and freshly grounded black pepper according to taste

Method

Add some water to a pan and add some salt to it. Bring it to a boil and add the florets to it. Cook for about 5 minutes and drain. In a small bowl, add garlic, vinegar, lemon juice, mustard, oil and red pepper flakes and whisk them together vigorously. Season with salt and pepper. Pour it over the broccoli and toss well. Keep it at room temperature for 10 minutes and then refrigerate for 1 hour. Serve it cold.

Enjoy!

Corn Salad with Italian Dressing

Ingredients

1 can Whole-kernel corn

1 cup Fresh tomato, chopped finely

1 cup Cucumber, peeled and chopped

½ cup Chopped celery

½ cup Green or sweet red pepper

2 Green onions

½ cup Italian salad dressing

Method

Place the corn into a bowl and add vegetables to it one by one. Toss it well. Pour the bottled Italian salad dressing and toss again. Cover it and refrigerate for several hours. Serve chilled.

Enjoy!

Asparagus and Bell Pepper Salad

Ingredients

1 ½ Fresh asparagus, trim off the ends and cut into small pieces

2 Yellow bell peppers, de-seeded and sliced

¼ cup Almond slices, toasted

1 Red onion

3 tbsp. Dijon mustard ¼ cup Olive oil ½ cup Parmesan cheese 3 cloves Garlic minced

2 tsp. Lime juice 2 tsp. Sugar 1 tsp. hot sauce Salad seasoning mix to taste

Method

Take a baking sheet and place the asparagus and bell peppers in a single layer. Sprinkle olive oil over the vegetables. Set 400 degrees F or 200 degrees C and preheat the oven. Place the baking sheet and roast it for 8-10 minutes. Turn the veggies occasionally. Cool and transfer the veggies in a large bowl. Add cheese, onion, roasted almonds. Whisk rest of the olive oil, mustard powder, sugar, hot sauce, lime juice, and salad seasoning. Sprinkle over the veggies and toss. Serve immediately.

Enjoy!

Tomato and Basil Salad

Ingredients

3 cups cooked rice

1 Cucumber, de-seeded and cubed

1 Red onion

2 Tomatoes

2 tbsp. Olive oil

2 tbsp. Cider vinegar

1 tsp. Fresh basil

¼ tsp. Pepper

½ tsp. Salt

Method

Take a large bowl and place the rice, cucumber, onion, tomatoes and toss them together. In a covered jar, combine olive oil, cider vinegar, basil together and mix vigorously. Add salt and pepper to taste. Sprinkle over the rice mixture and toss well. Refrigerate for several hours before serving.

Enjoy!

Colorful Garden Salad

Ingredients

5 tbsp. Red wine vinegar

3 tbsp. Grape seed oil

1/3 cup Chopped fresh cilantro

2 limes

1 tsp. White sugar2 cloves Garlic minced

1 packet Frozen shelled green soybeans

1 can Black beans

3 cups Frozen corn kernels

1 pint Cherry tomatoes divided into quarters

4 Green onions thinly sliced

¾ tsp. Salt

Method

Whisk the vinegar, oil, lime juice, cilantro, garlic, sugar, and salt together in a covered jar or large bowl to form a homogenous mixture. Keep it aside. Cook the soybean till they become nicely tendered. Cook the corn for 1 minute. Drain soybean and corn from water and transfer to a large bowl. Add the dressing. Toss it gently. Add tomatoes, onion to the mixture and toss. Cover the mixture. Refrigerate 2 to 4 hours. Serve chilled.

Enjoy!

Mushrooms Salad

Ingredients

1 pound Fresh mushrooms

1 Onion, finely sliced and separated into rings

Finely diced sweet red pepper, handful

2/3 cup Tarragon vinegar

½ cup Canola oil

1 tbsp. Sugar

1 garlic clove minced

Dash of hot pepper sauce

1 ½ tsp. Salt

2 tbsp. Water

Method

Add all the vegetables and other ingredients in a large bowl, except the red peppers, mushrooms and onion. Mix them well. Put mushrooms and onion to the mixture and toss gently till all the ingredients are evenly mixed. Cover the bowl and refrigerate overnight or 8 hours. Sprinkle red pepper over the salad before serving.

Enjoy!

Quinoa, Mint and Tomato Salad

Ingredients

1 ¼ cups Quinoa1/3 cup Raisins2 Tomatoes 1 Onion finely chopped

10 Radishes ½ Cucumber, 1/2, diced

2 tbsp. Sliced almonds slightly toasted

¼ cup Fresh mint chopped

2 tbsp. Fresh parsley finely chopped

1 tsp. Ground cumin¼ cup Lime juice2 tbsp. Sesame oil2 ½ cups Water Salt to taste

Method

Take a saucepan and add water and a pinch of salt to. Bring it to boil and add in the quinoa and raisins. Cover it and cook on simmer for 12-15 minutes. Remove it from heat and allow to cool. Drain quinoa and transfer to a bowl. In a medium sized bowl, combine onion, radish, cucumber, almonds, and tomatoes together. Toss it gently. Mix in the quinoa. Season it with spices, oil and herbs. Add salt to taste. Refrigerate for 2 hours. Serve chilled.

Enjoy!

Sauerkraut Salad Recipe

Ingredients

1 can Sauerkraut washed and drained well

1 cup Carrots grated

1 cup Green pepper finely chopped

1 jar Pimientos diced and drained

1 cup Celery thinly chopped

1 cup Onion thinly chopped

¾ cup Sugar

½ cup Canola oil

Method

Combine all the ingredients in a large bowl and mix well. Cover the bowl with a lid and refrigerate overnight or for 8 hours. Serve chilled.

Enjoy!

Quick Cucumber Salad

Ingredients

4 tomatoes, sliced into 8 wedges

2 large cucumbers nicely peeled and make fine slices

¼ cup Chopped fresh cilantro

1 large red onion, finely sliced

1 fresh lime, juiced

Salt to taste

Method

Place the sliced cucumbers, tomatoes, red onion, and cilantro in a large bowl and toss well. Add lime juice to the mixture and toss gently so that all the vegetables get coated with lime juice. Season the mixture with salt. Serve immediately or can be served after refrigeration.

Enjoy!

Tomato Slices with Creamy Dressing

Ingredients

1 cup Mayonnaise

½ cup Half-and-half cream

6 Tomatoes, sliced

1 Red onion cut thin into rings

¾ tsp. Dried basil

Few Lettuce leaves

Method

Combine mayonnaise and half-and-half cream together and whisk well. Add half the basil. Cover the mixture and refrigerate. Take a plate and line it with the lettuce leaves. Arrange the slices of tomatoes and onion rings. Drip the chilled dressing over the salad. Sprinkle then rest of the basils. Serve immediately.

Enjoy!

Beet Salad Platter

Ingredients

4 bunches Fresh small beets stems stripped off

2 heads Belgian endive

2 tbsp. Olive oil

1 pound spring lettuce mix

1 tbsp. Lemon juice

2 tbsp. White wine vinegar

1 tbsp. Honey

2 tbsp. Dijon mustard

1 tsp. Dried thyme

½ cup Vegetable oil

1 cup Crumbled feta cheese

Salt and pepper to taste

Method

Lightly coat the beet with vegetable oil. Roast for approximately 45 minutes in preheated oven, at 450 degrees F or 230 degrees C. Peel the beet and cut into small cubes. Combine lemon juice, mustard, honey, vinegar, and thyme in a blender and process it. Gradually add olive oil while the blender is running. Add salt and pepper to taste. In a salad bowl, place spring lettuce, enough amount of dressing and mix it well. Arrange endive on a plate. Pile the green salad. Top it with beet cubes and feta cheese.

Enjoy!

Chicken and Spinach Salad

Ingredients

5 cups Chicken cooked and cubed

2 cups Green grapes, cut into halves

1 cup Snow peas

2 cups Packed torn spinach

2 ½ cups Celery thinly sliced

7 Oz. cooked Spiral pasta or elbow macaroni

1 jar Marinated artichoke hearts

½ Cucumber

3 sliced Green onions with tops

Large spinach leaves, optional

Orange slices, optional

For Dressing:

½ cup Canola oil

¼ cup Sugar

2 tbsp. White wine vinegar

1 tsp. Salt

½ tsp. Dried minced onion

1 tsp. Lemon juice

2 tbsp. Minced fresh parsley

Method

Mix the chicken, peas, spinach, grapes, celery, artichoke heart, cucumber, green onion and cooked pasta in a large bowl and toss. Cover it and refrigerate for a few hours. Mix the other remaining ingredients in a separate bowl and refrigerate in a covered container. Prepare the dressing just before serving the salad by combining all the ingredients and whisking it well. Mix the components and toss well and serve immediately.

Enjoy!

German Cucumber Salad

Ingredients

2 large German cucumbers, sliced thinly

½ sliced Onions

1 tsp. Salt

½ cup Sour cream

2 tbsp. White sugar

2 tbsp. White vinegar

1 tsp. Dried dill

1 tsp. Dried parsley

1 tsp. Paprika Method

Arrange cucumbers and the rings of onion in a dish. Season the vegetables with salt and keep aside for at least 30 minutes. Squeeze out excess juice from cucumbers after marinating. Mix sour cream, vinegar, dill, parsley, and sugar in a vinegar, dill, and parsley together in a bowl. Coat cucumber and onion slices in this dressing. Refrigerate overnight or at least for 8 hours.

Just before serving, sprinkle paprika over the salad.

Enjoy!

Colorful Citrus Salad with Unique Dressing

Ingredients

1 can Mandarin oranges ¼ cup Fresh parsley finely chopped

Leaf lettuce, optional

½ Grapefruit peeled and sectioned

½ small Cucumber

1 small Tomato sliced

½ small Red onion

½ tsp. Brown sugar

3 tbsp. French or Italian salad dressing

1 tsp. Lemon juice

1 pinch dried tarragon

1 tsp. Dried basil

¼ tsp. Pepper

Method

Place the oranges in a small bowl after draining its juice and keep aside. Reserve the juice. Take a small bowl and add parsley, basil, tarragon, salad dressing, lemon juice, orange juice, brown sugar, and pepper. Whisk the mixture until smooth. Place lettuce leaves on a plate. Arrange the fruits one by one. Drizzle the dressing over the fruits and serve.

Enjoy!

Potato, Carrot and Beet Salad

Ingredients

2 Beets, boiled and sliced

4 Small potatoes, boiled and diced

2 Small carrots, boiled and sliced

3 Green onions, chopped

3 Small dill pickles, diced

¼ cup Vegetable oil

2 tbsp. Champagne vinegar

Salt to taste

Method

Combine all the ingredients and toss well to blend the flavors. Refrigerate for a few hours and serve chilled.

Enjoy!

Chicken Satay Healthier Healthy Salad Sammies

Ingredients

1 ½ bodyweight thin cut poultry various foods, cutlets

2 tbsp. vegetable oil

Grill planning, recommended: BBQ grill Mates Montreal Meal Seasoning by McCormick or rough sodium and pepper

3 rounded tbsp. large peanut butter

3 tbsp. black soy spices

1/4 cup any fruits juice

2 tsp. hot spices

1 lemon

1/4 seedless cucumber, cut into sticks

1 cup carrots cut into small pieces

2 cups lettuce leaves cut

4 crusty rolls, keisers or speakers, split

Method

Heat a BBQ grill pan or large non-stick package. Cover poultry in oil and BBQ grill planning and cook 3 minutes on each side in 2 batches.

Place peanut butter in a microwave safe dish and soften in the microwave on high for about 20 seconds. Mix soy, fruit juice, hot spices and lemon juice into the peanut butter. Throw poultry with satay spices. Mix the cut fresh vegetables. Place 1/4 of the fresh vegetables on sandwich bread and top with 1/4 Satay poultry mixture. Set the bun tops set up and offer or wrap for travel.

Enjoy!

Cleopatra's Chicken Salad

Ingredients

1 ½ chicken breasts

2 tbsp. extra-virgin olive oil

1/4 tsp. crushed red boost flakes

4 crushed garlic cloves

1/2 cup dry white wine

1/2 orange, juiced

A handful of sliced flat leaf parsley

Coarse sodium and black pepper

Method

Heat a large non-stick package over the stove. Add extra-virgin olive oil and heat. Add the crushed boost, crushed garlic cloves and chicken breasts. Sauté the chicken breasts until carefully browned on all sides, for about 5 to 6 minutes. Let the liquid cook out and tenders cook through, about 3 to 4 minutes more, and then remove the pan from heat. Press fresh squeezed lime juice over poultry and serve with parsley boost and salt as per taste. Serve immediately.

Enjoy!

Thai-Vietnamese salad

Ingredients

3 Latin lettuce, chopped

2 cups fresh vegetable seedlings, any variety

1 cup very perfectly sliced daikon or red radishes

2 cups peas

8 scallions, sliced on the bias

½ seedless cucumber, sliced in 1/2 lengthwise

1 pint yellow or red grape tomatoes

1 red onion, quartered and very perfectly sliced

1 selection of fresh excellent outcomes in, trimmed

1 selection fresh basil outcomes in, trimmed

2, 2-ounce packages sliced nut items, found on baking aisle

8 items almond toasted bread or anisette toasted bread, cut into 1-inch pieces

1/4 cup tamari black soy sauce

2 tbsp. vegetable oil

4 to 8 thin cut poultry cutlets, depending on size

Salt and fresh floor black pepper

1 lb. mahi mahi

1 ripe lime

Method

Combine all the ingredients in a large mixing bowl and serve chilled.

Enjoy!

Christmas Cobb Salad

Ingredients

Nonstick food preparation spray

2 tbsp. walnut syrup

2 tbsp. brownish sugar

2 tbsp. apple cider

1 lb. ham meal, fully ready, large dice

½ lb. bow tie grain, cooked

3 tbsp. sliced lovely gherkins

Bibb lettuce

½ cup sliced red onion

1 cup little diced Gouda

3 tbsp. sliced fresh parsley leaves

Vinaigrette, formula follows

Marinated Organic Beans:

1 lb. peas, decrease, cut in thirds

1 tsp. sliced garlic

1 tsp. red boost flakes

2 tsp. extra-virgin olive oil

1 tsp. white vinegar

Pinch salt

Black pepper

Method

Preheat the stove to 350 degrees F. Apply non-stick cooking spray to a baking dish. In a medium-sized dish, stir together the walnut syrup, brownish glucose, and the apple cider. Add the ham and mix well. Put the ham mixture on the baking dish and bake until warmed through and the ham develops color, about 20 to 25 minutes. Remove from the oven and set aside.

Add the grain, gherkins and parsley to the dish with the vinaigrette and stir to cover. Line a large offering dish with Bibb lettuce and add the grain. Organize the red onion, Gouda, marinated peas, and ready ham in rows on top of the grain. Serve.

Enjoy!

Green Potato Salad

Ingredients

7 to 8 scallions, cleaned, dried and cut into items, green and white-colored parts

1 little selection chives, sliced

1 tsp. Kosher salt

Freshly ground white pepper

2 tbsp. water

8 tbsp. extra-virgin olive oil

2 bodyweight red bliss celery, washed

3 bay leaves

6 tbsp. black vinegar

2 shallots, peeled, quartered lengthwise, sliced thin

2 tbsp. smooth Dijon mustard

1 tbsp. sliced capers

1 tsp. caper liquid

1 small bunch tarragon, chopped

Method

In a blender, blend together the scallions and chives. Season with salt as per taste. Add water and blend. Pour 5 tbsp. of the extra virgin olive oil through the top of the mixer in a slowly and blend until smooth. Bring the celery to a boil in a pot of water and reduce heat and simmer. Season the water with a touch of salt and add bay leaves in. Simmer the celery until they are tender when pierced with the tip of a blade, about 20 minutes.

In a dish large enough to hold the celery, stir together the black vinegar, shallots, mustard, capers and tarragon. Mix in the remaining extra virgin olive oil. Drain the celery and discard the bay leaves.

Place the celery in the dish and carefully grind them with the tines of a fork. Season carefully with boost and sodium and toss them well. Finish by adding the scallion and extra virgin olive oil mixture. Mix well. Keep heated at 70 degrees until serving.

Enjoy!

Burnt corn salad

Ingredients

3 sweet corn cobs

1/2 a cup of sliced onions

1/2 a cup of sliced capsicum

1/2 a cup of sliced tomatoes

Salt, to taste

For the salad dressing

2 tbsp. Olive oil

2 tbsp. Lemon juice

2 tsp. Chili powder

Method

The corn cobs are to be roasted over a medium heat until they are lightly burnt. After roasting them, the kernels of the corn cobs are to be removed with a help of a knife. Now take a bowl and mix the kernels, chopped onions, capsicum and tomatoes with salt and then keep the bowl aside. Now prepare the dressing of the salad by mixing the olive oil, lemon juice and chili powder and then chill it. Before serving, pour the dressing over the salad and then serve.

Enjoy!

Cabbage and grape salad

Ingredients

2 Cabbages, shredded

2 cups halved green grapes

1/2 cup finely chopped coriander

2 Green chilies, chopped

Olive oil

2 tbsp. Lemon juice

2 tsp. Icing Sugar

Salt and pepper, to taste

Method

To prepare the salad dressing take the olive oil, lemon juice with the sugar and salt and pepper in a bowl and mix them, well and then refrigerate it. Now, take the rest of the ingredients in another bowl, mix well and keep it aside. Before serving the salad, add the chilled salad dressing and mix them gently.

Enjoy!

Citrus salad

Ingredients

1 cup whole wheat pasta, cooked

1/2 a cup of sliced capsicum

1/2 cup carrots, blanched and chopped

1 green onion, shredded

1/2 cup oranges, cut in segments

1/2 cup sweet lime segments

1 cup bean sprouts

1 cup curd, low-fat

2-3 tbsp. of mint leaves

1 tsp. Mustard powder

2 tbsp. Powdered sugar

Salt, to taste

Method

To prepare the dressing, add the curd, mint leaves, mustard powder, sugar and salt in a bowl and mix them well until the sugar dissolves. Mix the rest of the ingredients in another bowl and then keep it aside to rest. Before serving add the dressing to the salad and serve chilled.

Enjoy!

Fruit and lettuce salad

Ingredients

2-3 Lettuce leaves, torn in pieces

1 Papaya, chopped

½ cup Grapes

2 Oranges

½ cup Strawberries

1 Watermelon

2 tbsp. Lemon juice

1 tbsp. Honey

1 tsp. Red chili flakes

Method

Take the lemon juice, honey and chili flakes in a bowl and mix them well and then keep aside. Now take the rest of the ingredients in another bowl and mix them well. Before serving, add the dressing to the salad and serve immediately.

Enjoy!

Apple and lettuce salad

Ingredients

1/2 a cup of muskmelon puree

1 tsp. Cumin seeds, roasted

1 tsp. Coriander

Salt and pepper to taste

2-3 Lettuce, torn in pieces

1 Cabbage, shredded

1 Carrot, grated

1 Capsicum, cut in cubes

2 tbsp. Lemon juice

½ cup Grapes, chopped

2 Apples, chopped

2 Green onions, chopped

Method

Take the cabbages, lettuce, grated carrots and capsicum to a pot and cover them with cold water and bring them to boil and cook them until they are cooked crisp, this can take up to 30 minutes. Now drain them and tie them in a cloth and refrigerate them. Now the apples are to be taken with the lemon juice in a bowl and refrigerate it. Now take the rest of the ingredients in a bowl and mix them properly. Serve the salad immediately.

Enjoy!

Bean and capsicum salad

Ingredients

1 cup Kidney beans, boiled

1 cup Chick peas, soaked and boiled

Olive oil

2 Onions, chopped

1 tsp. Coriander, chopped

1 Capsicum

2 tbsp. Lemon juice

1 tsp. Chili powder

Salt

Method

The capsicum is to be pierced with fork and then brush oil in them and then roast them over low heat. Now dip the capsicum in cold water and then the burnt skin is to be removed and then cut them in slices. Combine the rest of the ingredients with the capsicum and then mix them well. Before serving it, cool it for an hour or more.

Enjoy!!

Carrot and dates salad

Ingredients

1 ½ cup of carrot, grated

1 head of lettuce

2 tbsp. of almonds, roasted and chopped

Honey and lemon dressing

Method

Take the grated carrots in a pot of cold water and keep it for about 10 minutes, then drain it. Now the same is to be repeated with the head of lettuce. Now take the carrots and lettuce with other ingredients in a bowl and refrigerate it before serving. Serve the salad by sprinkling the roasted and chopped almonds over it.

Enjoy!!

Creamy pepper dressing for salad

Ingredients

2 cups of mayonnaise

1/2 a cup of milk

Water

2 tbsp. Cider vinegar

2 tbsp. Lemon juice

2 tbsp. Parmesan cheese

Salt

A dash of hot pepper sauce

A dash of Worcestershire sauce

Method

Take a large sized bowl, and take all the ingredients together in it and mix them well, so that no lump is found. When the mixture gets its desired creamy texture, pour it in your fresh fruit and veggie salad and then the salad with the salad dressing is ready to be served. This creamy and tangy dressing of pepper is not only well served with salads but can also be served with chicken, burgers and sandwiches.

Enjoy!

Hawaiian Salad

Ingredients

For orange dressing

A tbsp. of cornflour

About a cup of orange squash

1/2 a cup of orange juice

Cinnamon powder

For the salad

5-6 Lettuce leaves

1 Pineapple, cut in cubes

2 Bananas, cut in chunks

1 Cucumber, cut in cubes

2 Tomatoes

2 Oranges, cut in segments

4 Black dates

Salt, to taste

Method

For preparing the salad dressing, take a bowl and mix the cornflour in the orange juice and then add the orange squash to the bowl and cook it until the texture of the dressing thickens. Then the cinnamon powder and the chili powder are to be added to the bowl and then refrigerate it for few hours. Then prepare the salad, take the leaves of lettuce in a bowl and cover it with water for about 15 minutes. Now the sliced tomatoes are to be taken to a bowl with the pineapple chunks, apple, banana, cucumber and the segments of oranges in it with salt to taste and mix them well. Now add it to the lettuce leaves and then pour the chilled dressing over the salad, before serving.

Enjoy!!

Burnt corn salad

Ingredients

A pack of sweet corn cob

1/2 a cup of sliced onions

1/2 a cup of sliced capsicum

1/2 a cup of sliced tomatoes

Salt, to taste

For the salad dressing

Olive oil

Lemon juice

Chili powder

Method

The corn cobs are to be roasted over a medium heat until they are lightly burnt, after roasting them, the kernels of the corn cobs are to be removed with a help of a knife. Now take a bowl and mix the kernels, chopped onions, capsicum and tomatoes with salt and then keep the bowl aside. Now prepare the dressing of the salad by mixing the olive oil, lemon juice and chili powder and then chill it. Before serving, pour the dressing over the salad and then serve.

Enjoy!

Cabbage and grape salad

Ingredients

1 Cabbage head, shredded

About 2 cups of halved green grapes

1/2 a cup of finely chopped coriander

3 Green chilies, chopped

Olive oil

Lemon juice, to taste

Icing Sugar, to taste

Salt and pepper, to taste

Method

To prepare the salad dressing take the olive oil, lemon juice with the sugar and salt and pepper in a bowl and mix them, well and then refrigerate it. Now take the rest of the ingredients in another bowl and keep it aside. Before serving the salad, add the chilled salad dressing and mix them gently.

Enjoy!!

Citrus salad

Ingredients

About a cup of whole wheat pasta, cooked

1/2 a cup of sliced capsicum

1/2 a cup of carrots, blanched and chopped

Spring onion. Shredded

1/2 a cup of oranges, cut in segments

1/2 a cup of sweet lime segments

A cup of bean sprouts

About a cup of curd, low-fat

2-3 tbsp. of mint leaves

Mustard powder, to taste

Powdered sugar, to taste

Salt

Method

To prepare the dressing, add the curd, mint leaves, mustard powder, sugar and salt in a bowl and mix them well. Now mix the rest of the ingredients in another bowl and then keep it aside to rest. Before serving add the dressing to the salad and serve chill.

Enjoy!!

Fruit and lettuce salad

Ingredients

4 Lettuce leaves, torn in pieces

1 Papaya, chopped

1 cup Grapes

2 Oranges

1 cup Strawberries

1 Watermelon

½ cup Lemon juice

1 tsp. Honey

1 tsp. Red chili flakes

Method

Take the lemon juice, honey and chili flakes in a bowl and mix them well and then keep aside. Now take the rest of the ingredients in another bowl and mix them well. Before serving, add the dressing to the salad.

Enjoy!

Curry chicken salad

Ingredients

2 Skinless, boneless chicken breasts, cooked and cut into halves

3 - 4 Stalks of celery, chopped

1/2 a cup of mayonnaise, low in fat

2-3 tsp. of curry powder

Method

Take the cooked boneless, skinless chicken breasts with, the rest of the ingredients, celery, low fat mayonnaise, curry powder in a medium sized bowls and mix them properly. Thus this delicious and easy recipe is ready to be served. This salad can be used as stuffing of sandwich with lettuce over the bread.

Enjoy!!

Strawberry spinach salad

Ingredients

2 tsp. Sesame seeds

2 tsp. Poppy seeds

2 tsp. White sugar

Olive oil

2 tsp. Paprika

2 tsp. White vinegar

2 tsp. Worcestershire sauce

Onion, minced

Spinach, rinsed and torn in pieces

A quart of strawberries, chopped into pieces

Less than a cup of almonds, silvered and blanched

Method

Take a medium sized bowl; mix the poppy seeds, sesame seeds, sugar, olive oil, vinegar and paprika together with the Worcestershire sauce and onion. Mix them properly and cover it and then freeze it at least for an hour. Take another bowl and mix the spinach, strawberries and almonds together and then pour the herb mixture to it and then refrigerate the salad before serving for at least for 15 minutes.

Enjoy!

Sweet restaurant slaw

Ingredients

A 16 ounce bag of coleslaw mix

1 Onion, diced

Less than a cup of creamy salad dressing

Vegetable oil

1/2 a cup of white sugar

Salt

Poppy seeds

White vinegar

Method

Take a large sized bowl; mix the coleslaw mix and the onions together. Now take another bowl and mix together the salad dressing, vegetable oil, vinegar, sugar, salt and poppy seeds together. After mixing them well, add the mixture to the coleslaw mix and coat well. Before serving the delicious salad, refrigerate it for at least an hour or two.

Enjoy!

Classic macaroni salad

Ingredients

4 cups of elbow macaroni, uncooked

1 cup of mayonnaise

Less than a cup of distilled white vinegar

1 cup of white sugar

1 tsp. Yellow mustard

Salt

Black pepper, ground

A large sized onion, finely chopped

About a cup of carrots, grated

2-3 stalks of celery

2 Pimento peppers, chopped

Method

Take a large sized pot and take salted water in it and bring to boil, add the macaroni to it and cook them and let them cool for about 10 minutes and then drain it. Now take a large sized bowl and add the vinegar, mayonnaise, sugar, vinegar, mustards, salt and pepper and mix them well. When mixed well, add the celery, green peppers, pimento peppers, carrots and macaroni and again mix them well. After all the ingredients are mixed well, let it refrigerate for at least 4-5 hours before serving the delicious salad.

Enjoy!

Roquefort pear salad

Ingredients

Lettuce, torn on pieces

About 3-4 pears, peeled and chopped

A can of Roquefort cheese, shredded or crumbled

Green onions, sliced

About a cup of white sugar

1/2 a can of pecans

Olive oil

2 tsp. Red wine vinegar

Mustard, to taste

A clove of garlic

Salt and black pepper, to taste

Method

Take a pan and heat oil over a medium heat, then stir the sugar with the pecans in it and keep them stirring until the sugar is melted and the pecans get caramelized, and then let them cool. Now take another bowl and add the oil, vinegar, sugar, mustard, garlic, salt and black pepper and blend them well. Now mix the lettuce, pears, and blue cheese, avocado and green onions in a bowl and then add the dressing mixture to it and then sprinkle the caramelized pecans and serve.

Enjoy!!

Barbie's tuna salad

Ingredients

A can of white tuna

½ cup Mayonnaise

A tbsp. of parmesan style cheese

Sweet pickle, to taste

Onion flakes, to taste

Curry powder, to taste

Dried parsley, to taste

Dill weeds, dried, to taste

Garlic powder, to taste

Method

Take a bowl and add all the ingredients to it and mix well. Before serving, let them cool for an hour.

Enjoy!!

Holiday chicken salad

Ingredients

1 pound Chicken meat, cooked

A cup of mayonnaise

A tsp. of paprika

About two cups of cranberries, dried

2 Green onions, finely chopped

2 Green bell peppers, minced

A cup of pecans, chopped

Salt and black pepper, to taste

Method

Take a medium sized bowl, mix the mayonnaise, paprika and then season them to taste and add salt if needed. Now take the cranberries, celery, bell peppers, onions and nuts and mix them well. Now the cooked chicken is to be added and then mix them again well. Season them to taste and then if required add the ground black pepper to it. Before serving, let it cool for at least an hour.

Enjoy!!

Mexican bean salad

Ingredients

A can of black beans

A can of kidney beans

A can of cannellini beans

2 Green bell peppers, chopped

2 Red bell peppers

A pack of frozen corn kernels

1 Red onion, finely chopped

Olive oil

1 tbsp. Red wine vinegar

½ cup Lemon juice

Salt

1 Garlic, mashed

1 tbsp. Cilantro

1 tsp. Cumin, ground

Black pepper

1 tsp. Pepper sauce

1 tsp. Chili powder

Method

Take a bowl and mix the beans, bell peppers, frozen corn and red onions together. Now take another small sized bowl, mix the oil, red wine vinegar, lemon juice, cilantro, cumin, black pepper and then season to taste and add the hot sauce with the chili powder to it. Pour the dressing mix to it and mix well. Before serving, let them cool for about an hour or two.

Enjoy!!

Bacon ranch pasta salad

Ingredients

A can of uncooked tricolor rotini pasta

9-10 slices of bacon

A cup of mayonnaise

Salad dressing mix

1 tsp. Garlic powder

1 tsp. Garlic pepper

1/2 a cup of milk

1 Tomato, chopped

A can of black olives

A cup of cheddar cheese, shredded

Method

Take salted water in a pot and bring to boil. Cook the pasta in it until softens for about 8 minutes. Now take a pan and heat the oil in a pan and cook the bacons in it and when cook drain it and then chop it. Take another bowl and add the remaining ingredients to it and then add it with the pasta and bacons. Serve when mixed properly.

Enjoy!!

Red skinned potato salad

Ingredients

4 New red potatoes, cleaned and scrubbed

2 Eggs

A pound of bacon

Onion, finely chopped

A stalk of celery, chopped

About 2 cups of mayonnaise

Salt and pepper, to taste

Method

Take salted water to a pot and bring it to boil and then add the new potatoes to the pot and cook them for about 15 minutes, until tendered. Then drain the potatoes and let them cool. Now take the eggs to a pan and cover it with cold water and then bring the water to boil and then remove the pan from the heat and then keep it aside. Now cook the bacons and drain it and set it at a side. Now add and the ingredients with the potatoes and bacon and mix well. Chill it, and serve.

Enjoy!!

Black bean and couscous salad

Ingredients

A cup of couscous, uncooked

About two cups of chicken broth

Olive oil

2-3 tbsp. Lime juice

2-3 tbsp. Red wine vinegar

Cumin

2 Green onions, chopped

1 Red bell pepper, chopped

Cilantro, freshly chopped

A cup of frozen corn kernels

Two cans of black beans

Salt and pepper, to taste

Method

Boil the chicken broth and then stir the couscous, and cook it by covering the pan and then leave aside. Now mix the olive oil, lime juice, vinegar and cumin and then add the onions, pepper, cilantro, corn, beans and coat it. Now mix all ingredients together, and then before serving let it cool for few hours.

Enjoy!!

Greek chicken salad

Ingredients

2 cups of chicken meat, cooked

1/2 a cup of carrots, sliced

1/2 a cup of cucumber

About a cup of black olives, chopped

About a cup of feta cheese, shredded or crumbled

Italian-style salad dressing

Method

Take a large sized bowl, take the cooked chicken, carrots, cucumber, olives and cheese and mix them well. Now add the salad dressing mix to it and again mix them well. Now refrigerate the bowl, by covering it. Serve when chill.

Enjoy!!

Fancy chicken salad

Ingredients

½ cup Mayonnaise

2 tbsp. Cider vinegar

1 Garlic, minced

1 tsp. Fresh dill, finely chopped

A pound of cooked skinless and boneless chicken breasts

½ cup Feta cheese, shredded

1 Red bell pepper

Method

The mayonnaise, vinegar, garlic and dill are to be blended well and are to be refrigerated for at least 6-7 hours or overnight. Now the chicken, peppers, and cheese are to be stirred with it and then let it cool for few hours and then serve the healthy and delicious recipe of salad.

Enjoy!!

Fruity curry chicken salad

Ingredients

4-5 chicken breasts, cooked

A stalk of celery, chopped

Green onions

About a cup of golden raisins

Apple, peeled and sliced

Pecans, toasted

Green grapes, deseeded and halved

Curry powder

A cup of low fat mayonnaise

Method

Take a large sized bowl and take all the ingredients, like that of the celery, onions, raisins, sliced apples, toasted pecans, seedless green grapes with curry powder and mayonnaise to it and mix them well. When they are combined well with each other, let them rest for a few minutes and then serve the delicious and healthy chicken salad.

Enjoy!!

Wonderful chicken curry salad

Ingredients

About 4-5 skinless and boneless chicken breasts, cut in halves

A cup of mayonnaise

About a cup of chutney

A tsp. of curry powder

About a tsp. of pepper

Pecans, about a cup, chopped

A cup of grapes, deseeded and halved

1/2 a cup of onions, finely chopped

Method

Take a large sized pan, cook the chicken breasts in it for about 10 minutes and when cooked, tear it in to pieces with the help of a fork. Then drain them and let it cool. Now take another bowl, and add the mayonnaise, chutney, curry powder, and pepper and mix then together. Then stir the cooked and torn chicken breasts in the mix and then pour the pecans, curry powder and pepper in it. Before serving, refrigerate the salad for few hours. This salad is an ideal choice for burgers and sandwiches.

Enjoy!

Spicy carrot salad

Ingredients

2 Carrots, chopped

1 Garlic, minced

About a cup of water2-3 tbsp. Lemon juice

Olive oil

Salt, to taste

Pepper, to taste

Red pepper flakes

Parsley, fresh and chopped

Method

Take the carrots to the microwave and cook it for few minutes with the minced garlic and water. Take it out from the microwave, when the carrot is cooked and is softened. Then drain the carrots and set it aside. Now the lemon juice, olive oil, pepper flakes, salt and parsley are to be added to the bowl of carrots and mix them well. Let it cool for few hours and then the spicy delicious salad is ready to be served.

Enjoy!!

Asian apple slaw

Ingredients

2-3 tsp. Rice vinegar 2-3 tbsp. Lime juice

Salt, to taste

Sugar

1 tsp. Fish sauce

1 Julienned jicama

1 Apple, chopped

2 Scallions, finely chopped

Mint

Method

The rice vinegar, salt, sugar, lime juice and the fish sauce are to be mixed properly in a medium sized bowl. When they are mixed properly, the julienned jicamas are to be tossed with the chopped apples in the bowl and mix them well. Then the scallion chops and the mint are to be added and mixed. Before serving the salad with your sandwich or burger, let it cool for a while.

Enjoy!!

Squash and orzo salad

Ingredients

1 Zucchini

2 Scallions, chopped

1 Yellow squash

Olive oil

A can of cooked orzo

Dill

Parsley

½ cup Goat cheese, shredded

Pepper and salt, to taste

Method

The zucchini, chopped scallions with the yellow squash are to be sautéed in olive oil over medium heat. These are to be cooked for few minutes until they are softened. Now transfer them to a bowl and tip the cooked orzo in the bowl, with parsley, shredded goat cheese, dill, salt and pepper and then mix it again. Before serving the dish, cool the salad for few hours.

Enjoy!!

Salad with Watercress-fruit

Ingredients

1 Watermelon, cut into cubes

2 Peaches, cut into wedges

1 bunch Watercress

Olive oil

½ cup Lemon juice

Salt, to taste

Pepper, to taste

Method

The cubes of watermelon and the wedges of peaches are to be tossed together with the watercress in a medium sized bowl and then sprinkle the olive oil over it with the lime juice. Then season them to taste and if required add the salt and pepper, according to taste. When all the ingredients are easily and properly mixed, keep it aside or it can also be kept in the refrigerator for few hours and then the delicious to taste, yet healthy fruit salad is ready to be served.

Enjoy!!

Caesar Salad

Ingredients

3 Cloves of garlic, minced

3 Anchovies

½ cup Lemon juice

1 tsp. Worcestershire sauce

Olive oil

An egg yolk

1 head Romaine

½ cup Parmesan style cheese, shredded

Croutons

Method

The minced cloves of garlic with anchovies and lemon juice are to be pureed, then the Worcestershire sauce are to be added to it with the salt, pepper and yolk and then blend it again, until smooth. This blend is to be done with the help of a blender on a slow setting, now the olive oil is to be added slowly and gradually with it and then the romaine is to be tossed in it. Then the mixture is to be set aside for a while. Serve the salad with topping of parmesan cheese and croutons.

Enjoy!!

Chicken Mango Salad

Ingredients

2 Chicken breasts, boneless, cut in pieces

Mesclun greens

2 Mangoes, cut in cubes

¼ cup Lemon juice

1 tsp. Ginger, grated

2 tsp. Honey

Olive oil

Method

The lemon juice and honey is to be whisked in a bowl and then add the grated ginger to it and also add the olive oil to it. After mixing the ingredients in the bowl well, keep it aside. Then the chicken is to be grilled and then let it cool, and after cooling it tears the chicken in bite friendly cubes. Then take the chicken to the bowl and toss it well with the greens and the mangoes. After mixing all the ingredients well, keep it aside to cool then serve the delicious and interesting salad.

Enjoy!!

Orange salad with mozzarella

Ingredients

2-3 oranges, cut into slices

Mozzarella

Fresh basil leaves, torn in pieces

Olive oil

Salt, to taste

Pepper, to taste

Method

The mozzarella and the slices of orange are to be mixed together, with the fresh torn leaves of basil. After mixing them well, sprinkle the olive oil over it the mixture and season to taste. Then if required add salt and pepper, to taste. Before serving the salad, let the salad cool for few hours as this will give the salad the correct flavors.

Enjoy!!

Three-bean salad

Ingredients

1/2 a cup of cider vinegar

About a cup of sugar

A cup of vegetable oil

Salt, to taste

½ cup Green beans

½ cup Wax beans

½ cup Kidney beans

2 Red onions, finely chopped

Salt and pepper, to taste

Parsley leaves

Method

The cider vinegar with the vegetable oil, sugar and salt are to be taken in a pot and bring them to boil, then add the beans to it with the sliced red onions and then marinate it for at least an hour. After an hour, season to taste the salt, add salt and pepper, if required and then serve it with the fresh parsley.

Enjoy!!

Miso tofu salad

Ingredients

1 tsp. Ginger, finely chopped

3-4 tbsp. of miso

Water

1 tbsp. of rice wine vinegar

1 tsp. Soy sauce

1 tsp. Chili paste

1/2 a cup of peanut oil

A baby spinach, chopped

½ cup Tofu, cut in chunks

Method

The chopped ginger is to be pureed with miso, water, rice wine vinegar, soy sauce and chili paste. Then this mixture is to be blended with half a cup of peanut oil. When they are mixed properly, add the cubed tofu and the chopped spinach to it. Chill & serve.

Enjoy!!

Japanese radish Salad

Ingredients

1 Watermelon, cut in slices

1 Radish, sliced

1 Scallion

1 bunch Baby greens

Mirin

1 tsp. Rice wine vinegar

1 tsp. Soy sauce

1 tsp. Ginger, grated

Salt

Sesame oil

Vegetable oil

Method

Take the watermelon, radish with the scallions and green in a bowl and keep it aside. Now take another bowl, add the mirin, vinegar, salt, grated ginger, soy sauce with the sesame oil and the vegetable oil and then mix them well. When the ingredients in the bowl in mixed well, spread this mixture over the bowl of watermelons and radish. Thus the interesting yet very delicious salad is ready to be served.

Enjoy!!

Southwestern Cobb

Ingredients

1 cup Mayonnaise

1 cup Buttermilk

1 tsp. Hot Worcestershire sauce

1 tsp. Cilantro

3 Scallions

1 tbsp. Orange zest

1 Garlic, minced

1 head Romaine

1 Avocado, diced

Jicama

½ cup Sharp cheese, shredded or crumbled

2 Oranges, cut into segments

Salt, to taste

Method

The mayonnaise and the buttermilk are to be pureed with the hot Worcestershire sauce, scallions, orange zest, cilantro, minced garlic and salt. Now take another bowl and toss the romaine, avocados and the jicamas with oranges and the shredded cheese. Now pour the puree of the buttermilk over the bowl of oranges and keep it aside, before serving, so that the correct flavor of the salad is gained.

Enjoy!!

Pasta Caprese

Ingredients

1 packet Fusilli

1 cup Mozzarella, diced

2 Tomatoes, deseeded and chopped

Fresh leaves of basil

¼ cup Pine nuts, toasted

1 Garlic, minced

Salt and pepper, to taste

Method

The fusilli is to be cooked according to the instructions and then is to be kept aside to cool. After it is cooled, mix it with mozzarella, tomatoes, toasted pine nuts, minced garlic and basil leaves and season to taste, and add salt and pepper, if required, according to taste. Keep the whole mixture of the salad aside to cool and then serve it with your sandwiches or burgers or any of your meals.

Enjoy!!

Smoked-Trout Salad

Ingredients

2 tbsp. Cider vinegar

Olive oil

2 Shallots, minced

1 tsp. Horseradish

1 tsp. Dijon mustard

1 tsp. Honey

Salt and pepper, to taste

1 Can Smoked trout, flaked

2 apples, cut in slices

2 Beets, sliced

Arugula

Method

Take a large sized bowl and toss in it the flaked smoked trout with julienned apples, beets and arugula and then keep the bowl aside. Now take another bowl and mix the cider vinegar, olive oil, horseradish, minced shallots, honey and Dijon mustard and then season the mixture to taste and then if required add salt and pepper, according to your taste. Now take this mixture and pour over the bowl of julienned apples and mix well and then serve the salad.

Enjoy!!

Egg salad with Beans

Ingredients

1 cup Green beans, blanched

2 Radishes, sliced

2 Eggs

Olive oil

Salt and pepper, to taste

Method

The eggs are to be chard boiled at first and then mix it with the blanched green beans, sliced radishes. Mix them well, and then sprinkle over them olive oil and add salt and pepper, according to taste. When all the ingredients are mixed properly, keep it aside and let them cool. When the mix is cooled, the salad is ready to be served.

Enjoy!!

Ambrosia Salad

Ingredients

1 cup Coconut milk

2-3 slices Orange zest

A few drops Vanilla essence

1 cup Grapes, sliced

2 Tangerines, sliced

2 Apples, cut into slices

1 Coconut, grated and toasted

10-12 Walnuts, smashed

Method

Take a medium sized bowl and mix the coconut milk, orange zest with vanilla essence. When whisked properly add the sliced tangerine with the sliced apples and grapes. After mixing all the ingredients properly, refrigerate it for an hour or two, before serving the delicious salad. When the salad is cooled, serve the salad with sandwich or burgers.

Enjoy!!

Wedge salad

Ingredients

A cup of mayonnaise

A cup of blue cheese

1/2 a cup of buttermilk

A shallot

Lemon zest

Worcestershire sauce

Fresh leaves of parsley

Iceberg wedges

1 Egg, hard boiled

1 cup Bacon, crumbled

Salt and pepper, to taste

Method

The mayonnaise with the blue cheese, buttermilk, shallot, sauce, lemon zest and parsley are to be pureed. After making the puree, season it to taste and if required add the salt and pepper, according to taste. Now take another bowl and toss the iceberg wedges into the bowl with the egg mimosa, for making the egg mimosa stain the hard boiled eggs through the strainer. Now pour the mayo puree over the bowl of wedges and mimosa and then mix it well. The salad is to be served by spreading the fresh bacon over it.

Enjoy!!

Spanish pimiento salad

Ingredients

3 Scallions

4-5 Olives

2 Pimientos

2 tbsp. Sherry vinegar

1 head Paprika, smoked

1 head Romaine

1 handful Almonds

A clove of garlic

Bread slices

Method

The scallions are to be grilled and then are to be chopped in pieces. Now take another bowl and toss the pimientos and the olives in it with the almonds, smoked paprika, vinegar, romaine and the grilled and chopped scallions. Mix the ingredients of the bowl properly and keep it aside. Now the slices of the bread are to be grilled and when grilled the cloves of garlic are to be rubbed over the slices and then pour the mixture of the pimientos over the grilled breads.

Enjoy!!

Mimosa salad

Ingredients

2 Eggs, hard boiled

½ cup Butter

1 head Lettuce

Vinegar

Olive oil

Herbs, chopped

Method

Take a medium sized bowl and mix the lettuce, butter with the vinegar, olive oil and the chopped herbs. After mixing the ingredients of the bowl properly, keep the bowl aside for a while. In the meantime, the mimosa is to be prepared. For preparing the mimosa, the hard boiled eggs are to be peeled at first and then with a help of a strainer, strain the hard boiled eggs and thus the egg mimosa is ready. Now this egg mimosa is to be spooned over the bowl of salad, before serving the delicious mimosa salad.

Enjoy!!

Classic Waldorf

Ingredients

1/2 a cup of mayonnaise

2-3 tbsp. Sour cream

2 Chives

2-3 tbsp. Parsley

1 Lemon zest and juice

Sugar

2 Apples, chopped

1 stalk Celery, chopped

Walnuts

Method

Take a bowl and then the mayonnaise, sour cream is to be whisked with chives, lemon zest and juice, parsley, pepper and sugar. When the ingredients in the bowl are mixed properly keep it aside. Now take another bowl, and toss the apples, chopped celery and walnuts in it. Now take the mayo mixture and toss it with the apples and celery. Mix all the ingredients well, rest the bowl for a while and then serve the salad.

Enjoy!!

Black eyed pea salad

Ingredients

Lime juice

1 Garlic, minced

1 tsp. Cumin, ground

Salt

Cilantro

Olive oil

1 cup Black-eyed peas

1 Jalapeno, minced or smashed

2 Tomatoes, cut into dices

2 Red onions, finely chopped

2 Avocados

Method

The lime juice is to be whisked with the garlic, cumin, cilantro, salt and olive oil. When all these ingredients are properly mixed, toss this mixture with the smashed jalapenos, black eyed peas, avocados and the finely chopped red onions. When all the ingredients are mixed properly, give the salad a standing time for few minutes and then serve.

Enjoy!!

www.ingramcontent.com/pod-product-compliance
Lightning Source LLC
Chambersburg PA
CBHW071819080526
44589CB00012B/857